Living the Hope

Personal Story of Recovery and
Recovery Poems

Michael Roger

DEDICATION

For Mum – for believing in me and my story, for encouraging me, for supporting me continuously and for the unconditional love.
For my family – for putting up with me over the years and for supporting me and my journey of recovery despite the challenges that I go through daily.

CONTENTS

ACKNOWLEDGMENTS

To all the community support staff and peer support staff for believing in me and helping to write my story down. I would like to acknowledge the unending support from my mum, sister and the rest of the family in a challenging but rewarding journey. To all my friends thank you so much for your support over t he years.

1 JOURNEY OF RECOVERY

I was born in Wellington, New Zealand on 19 September 1958. I had an upset when I was eight years old as I was put back a class. I was very unhappy about it and became very unhappy as a child. I keep to myself and didn't tell anyone what was going on; I always felt like a misfit.

I over-studied for my School Certificate and was put on tranquilizers; however, I still passed four out of my five subjects: Geography (69%), Mathematics (68%), Bookkeeping (56%) and science (50%). I received 43% for English.

When I was 17, I left school and started working as a Trainee Lineman for Telecom (which was the Post Office until 1987) in May 1976. I did well at Telecom before I got sick. I went to the territorial's at the Army in Waiouru for 3-4 weeks, but unfortunately my back gave out; it became inflamed as I had Osteochondritis.

I passed the Trade Certificate in Telecommunications in 1979 (67%), which meant I became a Skilled Lineman in 1980. I then passed the Advanced Trade Certificate in 1981 (51%). I was never the brightest fish in town, I just tried hard.

MICHAEL ROGER

Three years and eight months after I first starting working at Telecom, I had a physical breakdown, which resulted in signs of mental illness eight months later. I was under extreme pressure from all parts of my life and would have gone down if I had stuck around. I was extremely lucky as I got a year's special leave in Telecom and shot overseas to Australia in 1981 by myself, where I knew no-one. I struck the right place at the right time at Telecom Australia in Melbourne. I lived for four months in Melbourne; I stayed in NSW and throughout Queensland, and I also travelled to Cairns and Sydney. It all went brilliantly. Telecom Australia said my "conduct, diligence and efficiency was judged most satisfactorily".

I got back to New Zealand and I couldn't have been any luckier, as I got a transfer on top of a year's special leave, where I went to Auckland, again knowing no-one. I lived and worked 15 months in Mt Albert and one month in Mt Eden, and then I broke. Miraculously, I got a second transfer to Wellington where I overcame a severe work trial, and then 15 months after I arrived back in Wellington, I went mad. I was 25 years old when I was first diagnosed with Schizophrenia.

I came off my medication at the end of that year, as I felt it was slowing me down too much and I might lose my job, and I didn't know any better. That is when things went bad and after one year back in the workforce, I ended up in Porirua hospital. However, I haven't made any more mistakes with my medication since.

At Porirua Hospital I met a nice male nurse who protected me from the old mental health system. He said "I'm going to protect you from the mental health system; we are going to talk about everything but mental illness", so I never got caught up in the old system. I never saw a Psychiatrist who would put my head through the grinder – I avoided the horrors of the old system. I have never been committed under the Mental Health Act.

4

Six months after being at Porirua Hospital, I went back to work. I was in a bad way but just got through it. I recuperated by the start of my second year back into work, where I was given a one-off chance by a Senior Foreman, acting as a Charge Hand. The following year, I was given another one-off chance by a Foreman to act as a Tradesman. The first two years of my illness after being in into psychosis. It meant that year was a very hard year working while I was becoming unwell. Around October, I pulled out of the workforce inches before I lost my sanity; however, I went back to work seven weeks later.

In September of 1989 (five years after first going into hospital), I was granted medical retirement, which I applied for. Telecom knew in the beginning there was something wrong in terms of my mental illness, so they were happy to approve it. A year later, Telecom became privatized and 80% of workers got axed, so it was good that I was granted medical retirement then because I would have been on the scrap heap like the rest of them. I got out while the job was still good.

The hardest thing for me was going back to work after losing my sanity, but it was actually the job that saved my bacon. Overall, I worked 13.5 years in Telecom – five years, eight months of that time I worked with schizophrenia. My lucky point was having a job in Telecom to go back too after I got sick; Telecom were good to me. I had a brilliant outcome when I came out of Telecom, which has left me with no loss or regrets. Although it is very rare for a schizophrenic to work 40-hours a week, I fought my illness as hard as you can fight it to do this. I think getting people with mental illnesses back into a normal job is important, as it gives you money, options, keeps you in society and gives you self esteem and a sense of purpose.

I remember I was at a church a year a half into my illness. I was traumatized; I couldn't sit still at all; I was right in the pit with excruciating mental pain. I walked out of this church on a sunny blue day – without a cloud in the sky – and there were three guys out on the field playing cricket and drinking beer, and I longed to be with them. Little did I know I would experience the euphoria of the social world six months later...

My social life was 100 times better after I got schizophrenia, as I was always tied up with singles dues and cabarets – which were absolutely, utterly brilliant. Whilst suffering from schizophrenia, I attended 114 singles dues and 74 cabarets, which is a big dance hall, with a great band and lots of people. Despite my schizophrenia, I found it easy to be sociable; the only thing I found easy after I got sick was attending singles dues and cabarets – I found that was easy as picking up a glass of water and drinking it. I pushed the happy bubble to the max. Throughout my time at the hospitals, I got on with 16 out of my 18 nurses. Socially, I was very bubbly and had a bubbly personality. I am an extrovert in nature and have never been called a show-off. I have remained positive all the way through.

In my second year back at work after the first hospital visit (1986), when I was in the pit and feeling sorry for myself, I started getting a hard time by a tradesman in my job. This was the only time I experienced stigma in the five years, eight months I worked with schizophrenia. This showed me the need for understanding for mentally ill people and what they are going through. We don't need pity (it's a bit of a putdown) – we need understanding. There are misconceptions all over the place with schizophrenia – Hollywood and the media. We are no more violent than anyone else. That all schizophrenics have split or multiple personalities is a misconception.

I have been on medication since being diagnosed with schizophrenia. About 12 years ago, I was getting my injection (for keeping my sanity) every three weeks. My illness meant that my concentration was damaged and I couldn't do academic work. I am fortunate in that I don't get hallucinations or delusions, but I do get disorganized thinking and motivation issues. I find simple things hard to do.

I find strength in the story of my life before and after I got sick; I find my optimism in what I achieved in my life and how lucky I was. For me, everyday is a good day. I like telling my story; I am continually at Take 5, where I talk to people and have coffee. I also like going to Oasis and connecting with people. Most people I have hung out with have been schizophrenics. I deal with my illness by talking about it every day – I think it's important to talk about your illness. A lot of people go into denial, which is the worst thing you can do.

I take my mental illness seriously. I believe schizophrenia is the worst mental illness and I fought my illness as hard as you can possibly fight it. It took a look of guts and tenacity. I didn't want to succumb to the illness. Mental illness is sharp and quick – and has to be acted on very quickly. It's all about doing it against adversity.

I am no better than anyone else – I have struck countless people with talents that suffer from schizophrenia but they have not had the opportunities that I've had; they have not been as lucky as I have been. Where I think I did best with my mental illness and functioned highly was socially, and my best achievements were in sports.

When I was 17, I left school and started working as a Trainee Lineman for Telecom (which was the Post Office until 1987) in May 1976. I did well at Telecom before I got sick. I went to the territorial's at the Army in Waiouru for 3-4 weeks, but unfortunately my back gave out; it became inflamed as I had Osteochondritis.

I passed the Trade Certificate in Telecommunications in 1979 (67%), which meant I became a Skilled Lineman in 1980. I then passed the Advanced Trade Certificate in 1981 (51%). I was never the brightest fish in town, I just tried hard.

Three years and eight months after I first starting working at Telecom, I had a physical breakdown, which resulted in signs of mental illness eight months later. I was under extreme pressure from all parts of my life and would have gone down if I had stuck around. I was extremely lucky as I got a year's special leave in Telecom and shot overseas to Australia in 1981 by myself, where I knew no-one. I struck the right place at the right time at Telecom Australia in Melbourne. I lived for four months in Melbourne; I stayed in NSW and throughout Queensland, and I also travelled to Cairns and Sydney. It all went brilliantly. Telecom Australia said my "conduct, diligence and efficiency was judged most satisfactorily".

I got back to New Zealand and I couldn't have been any luckier, as I got a transfer on top of a year's special leave, where I went to Auckland, again knowing no-one. I lived and worked 15 months in Mt Albert and one month in Mt Eden, and then I broke. Miraculously, I got a second transfer to Wellington where I overcame a severe work trial, and then 15 months after I arrived back in Wellington, I went mad. I was 25 years old when I was first diagnosed with schizophrenia.

I ended up in Ward 27 (Psychiatric Ward) in Wellington Hospital in 1984. It was my father who eventually took me in. The first time I went to hospital was hell. I was there for 6-7 weeks and then went straight back into 40-hour work weeks at Telecom from the hospital, as I would've been finished if I didn't get back to work. I was obsessed with my job and when I saw the guys working down the road in Telecom, I longed to be with them. I miraculously still had a job in Wellington to go back to after I left the hospital.

I came off my medication at the end of that year, as I felt it was slowing me down too much and I might lose my job, and I didn't know any better. That is when things went bad and after one year back in the workforce, I ended up in Porirua hospital. However, I haven't made any more mistakes with my medication since.

At Porirua Hospital I met a nice male nurse who protected me from the old mental health system. He said "I'm going to protect you from the mental health system; we are going to talk about everything but mental illness", so I never got caught up in the old system. I never saw a Psychiatrist who would put my head through the grinder – I avoided the horrors of the old system. I have never been committed under the Mental Health Act.

Six months after being at Porirua Hospital, I went back to work. I was in a bad way but just got through it. I recuperated by the start of my second year back into work, where I was given a one-off chance by a Senior Foreman, acting as a Charge Hand. The following year, I was given another one-off chance by a Foreman to act as a Tradesman. The first two years of my illness after being in Wellington Hospital (1984 – 1986) were particularly bad – I was in the pit. I was in excruciating mental pain and my self esteem was at rock bottom; however, I managed to bounce out of the hole I was in.

In September of the fourth year after I first went into hospital (1988), my head snapped under work pressure which meant another trip towards becoming very unwell. My internal brain cracked and I stated to go into psychosis. It meant that year was a very hard year working while I was becoming unwell. Around October, I pulled out of the workforce inches before I lost my sanity; however, I went back to work seven weeks later

In September of 1989 (five years after first going into hospital), I was granted medical retirement, which I applied for. Telecom knew in the beginning there was something wrong in terms of my mental illness, so they were happy to approve it. A year later, Telecom became privatized and 80% of workers got axed, so it was good that I was granted medical retirement then because I would have been on the scrap heap like the rest of them. I got out while the job was still good.

The hardest thing for me was going back to work after losing my sanity, but it was actually the job that saved my bacon. Overall, I worked 13.5 years in Telecom – five years, eight months of that time I worked with schizophrenia. My lucky point was having a job in Telecom to go back too after I got sick; Telecom were good to me. I had a brilliant outcome when I came out of Telecom, which has left me with no loss or regrets. Although it is very rare for a schizophrenic to work 40-hours a week, I fought my illness as hard as you can fight it to do this. I think getting people with mental illnesses back into a normal job is important, as it gives you money, options, keeps you in society and gives you self esteem and a sense of purpose.

I did well in sporting activities whilst suffering schizophrenia. Playing competition sport with my mental illness was very hard, but I was out there to win. When I was nearly finished working, I joined a C-grade competition tennis team in Wainuiomata. I hadn't played in 25 years but thought 'I've done quite a bit in my life, so I'll go and play sport', and joined up by myself. I became the top player in three weeks and even won runner up in the B- grade championship in tennis in 1988. I also won the Winter Social tennis championship; I was the top player and got nominated for the most improved player. A friend of mine asked me to join the darts club and in 1992, I played in the second division dart team in Wainuiomata. We won the second division and the second division peers. I was the first to get a 180 out of eight of us and I held the best peers record in the darts second division.

I remember I was at a church a year a half into my illness. I was traumatized; I couldn't sit still at all; I was right in the pit with excruciating mental pain. I walked out of this church on a sunny blue day – without a cloud in the sky –

and there were three guys out on the field playing cricket and drinking beer, and I longed to be with them. Little did I know I would experience the euphoria of the social world six months later.

My social life was 100 times better after I got schizophrenia, as I was always tied up with singles dues and cabarets – which were absolutely, utterly brilliant. Whilst suffering from schizophrenia, I attended 114 singles dues and 74 cabarets, which is a big dance hall, with a great band and lots of people. Despite my schizophrenia, I found it easy to be sociable; the only thing I found easy after I got sick was attending singles dues and cabarets – I found that was easy as picking up a glass of water and drinking it. I pushed the happy bubble to the max. Throughout my time at the hospitals, I got on with 16 out of my 18 nurses. Socially, I was very bubbly and had a bubbly personality. I am an extrovert in nature and have never been called a show-off. I have remained positive all the way though.

I lived with my family for 12 years after I got sick, and then I went and lived in the community for 13 years, eight months until my flat mate committed suicide. I moved to Richmond and was living there for near on five years. Now I live at the Wellink premises. I possibly suffered a stroke about four years ago, which has slowed me down. I have maintained a good relationship with my family throughout my illness – they don't treat me any differently; my father says "we treat LJ the same as anyone else". I think it is very important to have support from your family and after I stopping working, my life was dedicated to helping my family.

In my second year back at work after the first hospital visit (1986), when I was in the pit and feeling sorry for myself, I started getting a hard time by a tradesman in my job. This was the only time I experienced stigma in the five years, eight months I worked with schizophrenia. This showed me the need for understanding for mentally ill people and what they are going through. We don't need pity (it's a bit of a putdown) – we need understanding. There are misconceptions all over the place with schizophrenia – Hollywood and the media. We are no more violent than anyone else. That all schizophrenics have split or multiple personalities is a misconception.

I have been on medication since being diagnosed with schizophrenia. About 12 years ago, I was getting my injection (for keeping my sanity) every three weeks, I found that on the 2nd or 3rd day after I got the injection, I would go into a black mood for a couple of days. This went on for 18 months but fortunately, it naturally went away. That was the only time I suffered depression really. I have followed the pattern of taking my medication virtually perfectly. Schizophrenia is a serious condition and you have to take it seriously – it can be dangerous if you don't take your medication.

My illness meant that my concentration was damaged and I couldn't do academic work. I am fortunate in that I don't get hallucinations or delusions, but I do get disorganized thinking and motivation issues. I find simple things hard to do.

I find strength in the story of my life before and after I got sick; I find my optimism in what I achieved in my life and how lucky I was. For me, everyday is a good day. I like telling my story; I am continually at Take 5, where I talk to people and have coffee. I also like going to Oasis and connecting with people. Most people I have hung out with have been schizophrenics. I deal with my illness by talking about it every day – I think it's important to talk about your illness. A lot of people go into denial, which is the worst thing you can do.

I take my mental illness seriously. I believe schizophrenia is the worst mental illness and I fought my illness as hard as you can possibly fight it. It took a look of guts and tenacity. I didn't want to succumb to the illness. Mental illness is sharp and quick – and has to be acted on very quickly. It's all about doing it against adversity.

I am no better than anyone else – I have struck countless people with talents that suffer from schizophrenia but they have not had the opportunities that I've had; they have not been as lucky as I have been. Where I think I did best with my mental illness and functioned highly was socially, and my best achievements were in sports.

I have lived again despite my schizophrenia – I have had a second life. I have lived with no loss and no regrets, despite my illness. I did the best I could and now I live with contentment.

I think people with schizophrenia need to get on the right medication, need people to support them and need people to give them opportunities. It is all about pushing hope. My advice to fellow suffers is to get in touch with someone that is going to help you, count your blessings that there are people that can help, and keep on trying regardless of anything.

2 RECOVERY POEMS

I like to talk to people about my journey and I also like to share with people my life journey in poems. So here are some of the poems I have that focused on recovery from serious mental illness. I hope you will like them.

Recovery: Journey of Hope

The sun creates its own energy
and the stars brightness can
reach far and beyond
Their smiles never falter
Their life force never dim
Hope is like the sun and the stars
It's energy is self-creating
It's life energy can reach far and beyond
And its life force never diminished
It gives life to the afflicted and the despised
It rebuilds the self into fulfilment
Hope can be something personal
and can be build on other's hope
People's hope are diverse and
whatever hope you may have
Perhaps I may share with you what I know -
Hope is something that is truly Divine

Recovery: Journey of Discovery

I was willing
to ask for
direction
from friends
family
professionals.
but the path
of discovery is something
personal waiting
for me to
discover what
lies ahead.
I discovered
that recovery is
a journey
into the unknown.
A journey that
may be filled
with mystery and
awe alike. As I
travelled an unknown path
I discovered that
the most important thing
is to believe in oneself
and have hope.
And day by day,
as events unfold
one will discover
that the sun
had risen again.

Recovery: Journey of Self-Belief

I believe
that life
can experience
recovery
I believe
that life
can grow
I believe
in discovery
For I had
experience
all of them
All because
I have
self-belief
I believe
that life
can experience hope
I believe
in the power of love
I believe
 in the wisdom
 of experience
for I had
experience
all of them
All because I have self-belief
Yes I have belief in myself
And plenty of them.

Recovery: Journey of Love

LIVING THE HOPE

Life has
it's turns
       and twists
         When love
         is encountered and experienced
It turns the
inner self
        towards fulfilment
        and peace
Life has it's

 turns
       and twists
        Love is a force
that turns
death   into life
        Love is energy
        that
        untwists lives
that are tangled
It turns the inner
        self towards
           connectedness
           and wholeness
Life has
it's turns
       and twists
         When love meets
the soul and spirit
Something
        divine begins
           to happen
The soul begins
        to smile
The spirit begins
    to heal
For love

really is
the essence
of the Divine

LIVING THE HOPE

Believe
    that the sun
        will shine
            tomorrow
Even with
        clouds
           and the misty fog
And I may
      not see the
          sun's face
            in a cloudy day
but the sun
        will continue
           to shine
            even in the
darkest of days
        Growth is something
           that's within us
            A desire and a longing
Even with
      doubts and
        lack of belief
           The desire to be
better and grow
        is there always
           We may not
            see its face
But it continues
        to reside within us
           Recovery is a
            journey of growth
Even lingers the
        clouds of stagnation
           and lack of progress
            But growth is a
living seed
        Waiting to be

fed with love
and hope
And it will sprout
into the greatness of
a life that will
continue to grow
through recovery.

ABOUT THE AUTHOR

Michael Roger, which is a the author's pen name, lives in Wellington, New Zealand. He especially likes talking to people. He calls it 'talking therapy.' He is a very sociable person and he likes going for a walk to see his friends in the nearby area. He also likes dancing but he prefers to talk about his past dancing and social life and his past job and sports achievements which gives him hope and confidence in his recovery journey.